Keto Diet For Begginers

14-Day Ketogenic Diet Weight Loss Plan
with 28 Easy Low-Carb Recipes.

By:

Holly R.Evans

TABLE OF CONTENTS

INTRODUCTION

Anxious to lose some weight and looking for something that can burn fat at maximum speed? Have you tried endless other diet plans but nothing seems to work for more than a few weeks? For many people, the ketogenic diet is a great option for weight loss. It is very different and allows the person on the diet to eat a diet that consists of foods that you may not expect.

So the ketogenic diet, or keto, is a diet that consists of very low carbs and high fat. How many diets are there where you can start your day off with bacon and eggs, loads of it, then follow it up with chicken wings for lunch and then steak and broccoli for dinner. That may sound too good to be true for many. Well on this diet this is a great day of eating and you followed the rules perfectly with that meal plan.

When you eat a very low amount of carbs your body gets put into a state of ketosis. What this means is your body burns fat for energy. How low of an amount of carbs do you need to eat in order to get into ketosis? Well, it varies from person to person, but it is a safe bet to stay under 25 net carbs. Many would suggest that when you are in the "induction phase" which is when you are actually putting your body into ketosis, you should stay under 10 net carbs.

If you aren't sure what net carbs are, let me help you. Net carbs are the amount of carbs you eat minus the amount of dietary fiber. So if on the day you eat a total of 35 grams of net carbs and 13 grams of dietary fiber, your net carbs for the day would be 22.

WHAT IS THE KETO DIET?

The Keto diet involves going long spells on extremely low (no higher than 30g per day) to almost zero g per day of carbs and increasing your fats to a really high level (to the point where they may make up as much as 65% of your daily macronutrients intake.) The idea behind this is to get your body into a state of ketosis. In this state of ketosis the body is supposed to be more inclined to use fat for energy- and research says it does just this. Depleting your carbohydrate/glycogen liver stores and then moving onto fat for fuel means you should end up being shredded.

HOW DOES IT WORK?

The keto diet aims to force your body into using a different type of fuel. Instead of relying on sugar (glucose) that comes from carbohydrates (such as grains, legumes, vegetables, and fruits), the keto diet relies on ketone bodies, a type of fuel that the liver produces from stored fat.

Burning fat seems like an ideal way to lose pounds. But getting the liver to make ketone bodies is tricky:

- It requires that you deprive yourself of carbohydrates, fewer than 20 to 50 grams of carbs per day (keep in mind that a medium-sized banana has about 27 grams of carbs).

- It typically takes a few days to reach a state of ketosis.

- Eating too much protein can interfere with ketosis.

WHAT DO YOU EAT?

Because the keto diet has such a high fat requirement, followers must eat fat at each meal. In a daily 2,000-calorie diet, that might look like 165 grams of fat, 40 grams of carbs, and 75 grams of protein. However, the exact ratio depends on your particular needs.

Some healthy unsaturated fats are allowed on the keto diet — like nuts (almonds, walnuts), seeds, avocados, tofu, and olive oil. But saturated fats from oils (palm, coconut), lard, butter, and cocoa butter are encouraged in high amounts.

Protein is part of the keto diet, but it doesn't typically discriminate between lean protein foods and protein sources high in saturated fat such as beef, pork, and bacon.

What about fruits and vegetables? All fruits are rich in carbs, but you can have certain fruits (usually berries) in small portions. Vegetables (also rich in carbs) are restricted to leafy greens (such as kale, Swiss chard, spinach), cauliflower, broccoli, Brussels sprouts, asparagus, bell peppers, onions, garlic, mushrooms, cucumber, celery, and summer squashes. A cup of chopped broccoli has about six carbs.

KETO RISKS

A ketogenic diet has numerous risks. Top of the list: it's high in saturated fat. McManus recommends that you keep saturated fats to no more than 7% of your daily calories because of the link to heart disease. And indeed, the keto diet is associated with an increase in "bad" LDL cholesterol, which is also linked to heart disease.

Other potential keto risks include these:

Diarrhea

If you find yourself running to the bathroom more often while on a ketogenic diet, a quick internet search will show you that you're not alone. (Yes, people are tweeting about keto diarrhea.) This may be due to the gallbladder—the organ that produces bile to help break down fat in the diet—feeling "overwhelmed," says Axe.

Diarrhea can also be due to a lack of fiber in the diet, says Kizer, which can happen when someone cuts way back on carbs (like whole-grain bread and pasta) and doesn't supplement with other fiber-rich foods, like vegetables. It can also be caused by an intolerance to dairy or artificial sweeteners—

things you might be eating more of since switching to a high-fat, low-carb lifestyle.

Nutrient deficiency.

"If you're not eating a wide variety of vegetables, fruits, and grains, you may be at risk for deficiencies in micronutrients, including selenium, magnesium, phosphorus, and vitamins B and C," says registered dietitian Kathy McManus, director of the Department of Nutrition at Harvard-affiliated Brigham and Women's Hospital.

Liver problems. With so much fat to metabolize, the diet could make any existing liver conditions worse.

Kidney problems.

The kidneys help metabolize protein, and McManus says the keto diet may overload them. (The current recommended intake for protein averages 46 grams per day for women, and 56 grams for men).

Less Muscle Mass, Decreased Metabolism

Another consequence of keto-related weight changes can be a loss of muscle mass, says Kristen Kizer, RD, a nutritionist at Houston Methodist

Medical Center.—especially if you're eating much more fat than protein. "You'll lose weight, but it might actually be a lot of muscle," she says, "and because muscle burns more calories than fat, that will affect your metabolism."

When a person goes off the ketogenic diet and regains much of their original weight, it's often not in the same proportions, says Kizer: Instead of regaining lean muscle, you're likely to regain fat. "Now you're back to your starting weight, but you no longer have the muscle mass to burn the calories that you did before," she says. "That can have lasting effects on your resting metabolic rate, and on your weight long-term."

Constipation

The keto diet is low in fibrous foods like grains and legumes.

Fuzzy thinking and mood swings

"The brain needs sugar from healthy carbohydrates to function. Low-carb diets may cause confusion and irritability," says McManus.

HOW TO LOSE OVER 25LBS IN 8 WEEKS WITHOUT HARMFUL EXERCISES AND TO SAVE OVER 100$/WEEK

Although exercise can certainly help build fat-burning muscle and maintain a svelte physique, it won't shrink your waistline as much as changing your diet will. So now that we know "eating less" should take priority in your weight-loss journey, where to start? Because it's easier said than done, we've uncovered slimming secrets that can help you tackle your muffin top through diet swaps as well as lifestyle and eating habit changes.

Check this out how you can avoid becoming a gym rat below, and then double down on your efforts by with healthy recipes, supermarket shopping guides, and essential nutrition tips delivered to your doorstep.

Refrain from Alcohol

Cut down your alcohol and sugar consumption, and limit saturated and trans fats, as these can wreak havoc on your weight-loss efforts and your health. Avoid sugar from desserts, fruits in syrup, and soda. Steer clear of unhealthy fats, which are present in baked and fried foods, hard margarine, lard, fatty meats and full-fat dairy products. Choose healthy fats from olive or canola oil and soft margarine instead.

Eat Healthy Fats

When you're trying to lose weight, the last thing you want to do is eat anything fatty, right? Wrong. You just have to make sure you're eating the right kind of fat. While eating certain types of fat are definitely no-nos when you're trying to lose weight — looking at you, saturated fat! — adding healthy fats into your diet is a game-changer. Research has shown eating good-for-you fats like avocado on a daily basis — even if that's just throwing some onto your salad for lunch — can leave you so full and satisfied that you're not reaching for unhealthy, sugary snacks later on. And without all those excess calories, you're bound to drop unwanted weight.

Hop on the Yoga Bandwagon

You might not see yoga as a solid weight-loss method, but think again. Aside from working out every muscle in your body and reducing your stress levels, you're also raising your heart rate to reap some major fat-burning benefits. Try this workout that's designed to help you drop pounds and tone up in process.

Dance the Weight Off

The best types of workouts are the ones you're having so much fun during that you forget you're even working out in the first place. If you want to lose weight, try this 35-minute by Body by Simone creator Simone de la Rue. You'll be sweating in no time.

Increase Your H20 Intake

Here's your permission to dump that electric-green juice craze down the drain. A better plan is to sip water throughout the day. Research shows it actually helps you cut down on calories. Often, thirst is confused for hunger. And try salt water, while you're at it. When it comes to H20, salt is not the enemy. "Water needs electrolytes like sodium, potassium, and chloride to be best absorbed," says Jenny Westerkamp, an R.D. in Chicago, which explains why they're added to popular sports drinks.

She recommends adding a pinch of Celtic sea salt or real salt (unrefined and unbleached) to your water before chugging. "The electrolytes in the salt will push water into the cells where they need to be, rather than letting the water get flushed out, causing you to go to the bathroom every other minute." You'll notice a spike in energy after staying hydrated, too, and you'll be less likely to give in to cravings which are even harder to avoid when you're running on empty.

Rethink What "Exercise" Really Means

We know we said these tips were about shedding pounds without working out, but being active is important, so here's radical idea: Change the way you think about exercise by choosing to do something you enjoy. "It doesn't have to be in a gym," Christy Harrison, a Brooklyn-based dietitian, says. "It could be a dance class or going for a run around your neighborhood." And it might even be worth it to get into tree pose when you've only got a few minutes. A study published in the journal PLOS ONE found that just 10 minutes of exercise has huge health benefits.

Give Meal-Prepping a Try

Yeah, yeah — meal-prepping isn't exciting. That's nothing new. But by spending a few hours every weekend preparing some meals for the week ahead, you could see a lot of progress in a short amount of time. Plus, you'll save money by cutting back on the delivery. "When you plan an entire week of dinner in advance, you're way less likely to go off course and indulge in foods that aren't good for you," says Pamela Salzman, a certified holistic health expert and cooking instructor. Start with making your lunches in advance and go from there.

Get Smart About Nutrition

Crying tears of sugar because you ate a donut that isn't on your approved list of foods isn't going to do you any good. You ate a donut. Cool. Move on. Here's why: Remember when you were a kid and your mom banned soda from your life forever and it only led to serious root beer binges when you got to your friend's house? Those same rules are in play here. Get label-crazed and you'll lose your mind — not excess weight. And cutting yourself off from all of your favorite things will only lead to overdoing it on the sugary, salty foods.

Instead, Harrison, says. you should look at foods as a way of self-care — eat what makes you feel good and forget about it as a means of slimming down (although a solid side effect of healthy eating: weight loss). Does that mean a free-for-all on the candy bowl? No. But it's a rule your body will naturally adapt to, not something you have to force on it. A bowl of almonds made you feel amazing in the mid-afternoon sales meeting, but those red gummies, not so much. Next time, you'll likely reach for the almonds.

BEST KETO-FRIENDLY DRINKS

If you're on a ketogenic diet, you're super focused on what you're eating and especially what you're not eating. But don't forget that what you sip can set you up for success, too.

Bear in mind, that going Keto means you can't have alcohol, right? Here's a list of Keto Friendly drinks

Water Is the Best Drink You Can Sip on the Keto Diet

This is hands down the best drink for you — keto or not, says Keene. Keep a water bottle near you at all times and sip throughout the day to stay ahead of your hydration.

Tea

Tea is another great option for keto, and if you don't add anything to it, it's perfectly keto-friendly, too. There are a lot of different tea varieties, and if you're new to tea, we recommend experimenting with a few types to find out what you like the most.

Black Tea

This is the strongest, and usually has the highest caffeine content. Similarly to coffee, there are a lot of different kinds of black teas out there – there are lots of different sorts of tea, from different countries of origin (Indian black tea, such as Assam and Darjeeling being one of the most popular ones, for example), with different flavours, and so on.

Green Tea

This is also extremely popular and readily available in almost any supermarket or health food store around the world.

Seltzer or Sparkling Water Is Another Carb-Free Drink Option

This is a great way to mix up your usual water — just avoid tonic, which looks like clear, plain bubbled water, but actually contains a ton of sugar. Adding a squeeze of lemon adds nearly ½ gram (g) of carbohydrates, notes the U.S. Department of Agriculture (USDA).

Plain Coffee, or Coffee With Unsweetened Heavy Cream, Is Also Okay on the Keto Diet

Like with tea, it's what you add to your brew that matters most. Drinking it black is completely calorie free, but many keto dieters will appreciate the added fat that heavy cream provides, says Scott Keatley, RDN, of Keatley Medical Nutrition Therapy in New York City. For adults, up to 400 milligrams (mg) per day of caffeine is considered safe, according to the Mayo Clinic. For reference, 1 cup — 8 fluid ounces (oz) — of coffee contains about 92 mg, per the USDA, while a tall coffee at Starbucks contains 245 mg, according to the company website.

Diet Soda

Like soda, but without the sugar and the calories.

Juice Alternatives

There are also some low-calorie and zero calorie drinks like Powerade Zero and Vitamin Water Zero that taste good and hydrate you without the extra sugar. Just make sure you read the labels of any tasty low-calorie drink you buy because they may have added sugars.

Low-Carb Dairy Products and Dairy Alternatives

A little bit of milk in your coffee or tea is okay, but don't have too much. If you need to use more than a couple of tablespoons of milk, try using heavy cream or a dairy alternative like unsweetened coconut milk or almond milk instead.

Energy Drinks

Most energy drinks are packed with more sugar than soda, but there are many low-carb and zero carb energy drinks on the market. However, just because it says "low-carb" on the container doesn't mean that it will fit within your daily carb limit. Always read labels carefully, especially when you are purchasing energy drinks.

Bone Broth Can Be a Comforting Keto-Friendly Drink

There's something uniquely warming and comforting about sipping a steaming cup of bone broth. One brand notes this liquid offers 0 carbs and 1 cup contains less than 50 calories while adding 9 g of protein. Traditional broth is a stellar option, too, though it has less protein. One cup contains 13 calories and 2.5 g of protein, according to the USDA.

Nut Milks Are Also Low-Carb and Okay for Keto Dieters

Almond, coconut, and cashew milks make for great choices if you want to mix things up, as they contain 1 g (or less) of carbs per cup. Just be sure to always read the nutrition label closely and choose unsweetened varieties. These are often fortified with vitamins and minerals, so they're a good way to get in calcium and vitamin D.

THE 7 IMPORTANT THINGS YOU SHOULD KNOW ABOUT THE KETO DIET BEFORE YOU START

The keto diet has go vira in popularity, and it's because going keto has helped celebrites like Gwyneth Paltrow, Halle Berry, Kim Kardashian used Keto to transform their bodies and many people to lose their weight, in some cases more than 150 pounds. But the diet, which is high in fat, is also controversial, as dietitians worry about the implications of cutting out an entire food group (grains and carbs) and eating an abundance of saturated fat.

But if you're curious about embarking on the keto diet, here's everything you need to know before getting started.

Keto is more than a diet.

It's a way of eating (WOE). You'll often hear people describe their keto diet as a "lifestyle" or "way of eating." That's because it's not something you can stop and start like most other diets. In fact, going on and off keto can mess up your metabolism and confuse your body, possibly causing you to gain more weight. For keto to be effective in enhancing your health, helping you lose weight, and improving your mental focus and energy levels, you must be consistent and make it a permanent lifestyle change.

Keto requires time.

You'll hear about keto success stories where weight starts to melt off almost immediately. Those cases are typically associated with people who have lots of weight to lose. In general, the more weight you have to lose, the faster it'll come off at the beginning. Another thing to keep in mind is that slow and steady weight loss is healthier, more sustainable, and more likely to stay off. So be patient with yourself. Don't give up on the keto diet because you don't immediately see drastic weight loss.

Keto can be customized.

The ketogenic diet – generally speaking – is 75% fat, 20% protein, 5% carbohydrates. But daily carb intake can vary from 20 grams to 50 grams depending on how your body processes carbs. There's no magic number of carbs that'll get you into ketosis. If you're not losing weight or unable to get into ketosis at 50 grams, keep dropping your carb macros until you achieve the results you want. Bottom line: do what works for you.

Going keto can impact your workouts.

You may lose some strength and endurance at the beginning of your keto diet. This is because your body is used to burning carbs for fuel, and it suddenly doesn't have that option anymore. As it adjusts to burning fat, you'll notice that your workout capacity will return to normal. And you may even notice that your athletic performance improves once your body is fully keto-adapted and burning fat for fuel.

Stick With It

After that initial shedding period, the weight loss may slow significantly. But that's ok. As your body gets used to the diet you'll likely lose weight over time—which is actually healthier and more sustainable than losing a lot of weight overnight.

Stay Hydrated

Since you lose a lot of water weight on Keto, especially at first, it's crucial to drink a lot of water to stay hydrated. Drink more than you are used to as you are changing the way your body is functioning. Increase your salt intake as well to help retain water and prevent dehydration (a common side effect of the diet).

The biggest mistake people make while on Keto, you can avoid this

Eating Too Much Protein

To some of you, this may not seem like such a bad thing. You aren't allowed many carbs so a way to supplement that is through consuming protein.

However, having too much protein is going to have negative effects on your body during a keto diet.

Your body only needs so much protein, anything more than that and it starts to get converted into fat. We are trying to eliminate fat so anything that adds fat to your body is a negative.

Avoiding this is pretty simple. All you need to do is focus on your macros. Stay with your macros and you won't have to worry about having anything in excess. You will only have exactly what you need.

KETO DIETING? HERE ARE 10 FOODS YOU MUST HAVE IN YOUR KITCHEN

Because we are surrounded by fast food restaurants and processed meals, it can be a challenge to avoid carb-rich foods, but proper planning can help.

Plan menus and snacks at least a week ahead of time, so you aren't caught with only high carb meal choices. Research keto recipes online; there are quite a few good ones to choose from. Immerse yourself in the keto lifestyle, find your favorite recipes, and stick with them.

There are a few items that are staples of a keto diet. Be sure to have these items on hand:

- **Eggs** - Used in omelets, quiches (yes, heavy cream is legal on keto!), hard boiled as a snack, low carb pizza crust, and more; if you like eggs, you have a great chance of success on this diet
- **Bacon** - Do I need a reason? breakfast, salad garnish, burger topper, BLT's (no bread of course; try a BLT in a bowl, tossed in mayo)

- **Cream cheese** - Dozens of recipes, pizza crusts, main dishes, desserts
- **Shredded cheese** - Sprinkle over taco meat in a bowl, made into tortilla chips in the microwave, salad toppers, low-carb pizza and enchiladas
- **Lots of romaine and spinach** - Fill up on the green veggies; have plenty on hand for a quick salad when hunger pangs hit
- **EZ-Sweetz liquid sweetener -** Use a couple of drops in place of sugar; this artificial sweetener is the most natural and easiest to use that I've found
- **Cauliflower** - Fresh or frozen bags you can eat this low-carb veggie by itself, tossed in olive oil and baked, mashed in fake potatoes, chopped/shredded and used in place of rice under main dishes, in low-carb and keto pizza crusts, and much more
- **Frozen chicken tenders** - Have a large bag on hand; thaw quickly and grill, saute, mix with veggies and top with garlic sauce in a low carb flatbread, use in Chicken piccata, chicken alfredo, tacos, enchiladas, Indian Butter chicken, and more
- **Ground beef** - Make a big burger and top with all sorts of things from cheese, to sauteed mushrooms, to grilled onions... or

crumble and cook with taco seasoning and use in provolone cheese taco shells; throw in a dish with lettuce, avocado, cheese, sour cream for a tortilla-less taco salad

- **Almonds (plain or flavored)** - these are a tasty and healthy snack; however, be sure to count them as you eat, because the carbs DO add up. Flavors include habanero, coconut, salt and vinegar and more.

28 CHEEP, TASTY KETO FRIENDLY RECIPIES

The Ketogenic diet trend has already given us some amazing new ways to enjoy our food and we aren't going to lie, we are loving every minute of it! Is the Keto diet right for you?

Here are Keto Friendly recipies you can try in the kitchen or order in your favourite restaurants. You can still out to eat with your friends.

BreakFast

Keto Chicken Parmesan

"A delicious keto-friendly chicken Parmesan. Enjoy a classic Italian dish, and keep your macros in check!"

Ingredients

2 servings
442 cals
Prep: 20 m
Cook: 8 m
Total: 28

- 1 (8 ounce) skinless, boneless chicken breast
- 1 egg
- 1 tablespoon heavy whipping cream
- 1 1/2 ounces pork rinds, crushed
- 1 ounce grated Parmesan cheese
- 1/2 teaspoon salt
- 1/2 teaspoon garlic powder
- 1/2 teaspoon red pepper flakes (optional)
- 1/2 teaspoon ground black pepper

- 1/2 teaspoon Italian seasoning
- 1/2 cup jarred tomato sauce (such as Rao's®)
- 1/4 cup shredded mozzarella cheese
- 1 tablespoon ghee (clarified butter)
- Add all ingredients to list

Instructions

- Set oven rack about 6 inches from the heat source and preheat the oven's broiler.
- Slice chicken breast through the middle horizontally from one side to within 1/2 inch of the other side. Open the two sides and spread them out like an open book. Pound chicken flat until about 1/2-inch thick.
- Beat egg and cream together in a bowl.
- Combine crushed pork rinds, Parmesan cheese, salt, garlic powder, red pepper flakes, ground black pepper, and Italian seasoning in bowl; transfer breading to a plate.
- Dip chicken into egg mixture; coat completely. Press chicken into breading; thickly coat both sides.
- Heat a skillet over medium-high heat; add ghee. Place chicken in the pan; cook until no

longer pink in the center and the juices run clear, about 3 minutes per side. An instant-read thermometer inserted into the center should read at least 165 degrees F (74 degrees C). Be careful to keep breading in place.

- Transfer chicken to a baking sheet. Cover with tomato sauce; top with mozzarella cheese.
- Broil until cheese is bubbling and barely browned, about 2 minutes.

Nutrition

Serving Size: 1 Calories: 509 Fat: 28g Carbohydrates: 10.5g Fiber: 6g

Keto mushroom omelet

Looking for a quick and easy way to start your day? This hearty omelet is super healthy, and just takes a few minutes to make! Fresh mushrooms make a delicious filling. Enjoy this keto meal anytime

Time: 5 + 10 m
kcal: 510

Ingredients

- 3 eggs
- 1 oz. butter, for frying
- 1 oz. shredded cheese
- 1/5 yellow onion
- 3 mushrooms
- salt and pepper

Instructions

- Crack the eggs into a mixing bowl with a pinch of salt and pepper. Whisk the eggs with a fork until smooth and frothy.
- Add salt and spices to taste.
- Melt butter in a frying pan. Once the butter has melted, pour in the egg mixture.

- When the omelet begins to cook and get firm, but still has a little raw egg on top, sprinkle cheese, mushrooms and onion on top (optional).
- Using a spatula, carefully ease around the edges of the omelet, and then fold it over in half. When it starts to turn golden brown underneath, remove the pan from the heat and slide the omelet on to a plate.

Recipe Note!

Serve the omelet with a crispy, green salad with vinaigrette dressing on the side. Yum!

Nutrition Info
Net carbs: 3 % (4 g)
Fiber: 1 g
Fat: 77 % (43 g)
Protein: 20 % (25 g)
kcal: 510

Keto Pancakes

There's nothing like a big stack of pancakes for breakfast—they're a breakfast staple! Just because you're on the Keto diet doesn't mean you've gotta miss out on the joys of flapjacks. This recipe is super easy and will definitely satisfy your craving.

Yields: 10
Prep Time: 0 hours 5 mins
Total Time: 0 hours 15 mins

Ingredients

- 1/2 c. almond flour
- 4 oz. cream cheese, softened
- 4 large eggs
- 1 tsp. lemon zest
- Butter, for frying and serving

Instructions

- In a medium bowl, whisk together almond flour, cream cheese, eggs, and lemon zest until smooth.

- In a nonstick skillet over medium heat, melt 1 tablespoon butter. Pour in about 3 tablespoons batter and cook until golden, 2 minutes. Flip and cook 2 minutes more. Transfer to a plate and continue with the rest of the batter.
- Serve topped with butter.

Recipe Note
Total recipe yields 4-6 small pancakes.

Nutrition Facts
Calories 339 Calories from Fat 270
Potassium 145mg 4%
Total Carbohydrates 7g 2%
Dietary Fiber 3g 12%
Sugars 1g
Protein 12g 24

Keto Banana Nut Muffins

Tired of eggs for keto breakfast? These Keto Banana Nut Muffins are so simple and delicious, your kids will love helping you make them on the weekends just as much as they'll love helping you eat them!

Prep Time: 10 Minutes
Cook Time: 20 Minutes
Total Time: 30 minutes
Yield: 10 Muffins

Ingredients

Muffin Battter

- 1 1/4 Cup almond flour (I use this)
- 1/2 Cup powdered erythritol (I use this)
- 2 tablespoons ground flax (feel free to omit if you don't have it...it just adds a bit more depth to the flavors)
- 2 teaspoons baking powder
- 1/2 teaspoons ground cinnamon
- 5 tablespoon butter, melted
- 2 1/2 teaspoons banana extract
- 1 teaspoon vanilla extract
- 1/4 cup unsweetened almond milk

* 1/4 cup sour cream
* 2 eggs

Walnut Crumble

* 3/4 cup chopped walnuts
* 1 tablespoon butter, cold and cut in 4 pieces
* 1 tablespoon almond flour
* 1 tablespoon powdered erythritol

Instructions

* Preheat oven to 350

* Prepare muffin tin with 10 paper liners, and set aside

* In a large bowl, mix almond flour, erythritol (or preferred sweetener) flax, baking powder and cinnamon

* Stir in butter, banana extract, vanilla extract, almond milk, and sour cream.

* Add eggs to mixture and gently stir until fully combined.

- Fill muffin tins about 1/2-3/4 full with mixture.

- **If you need more accurate measurements, weigh the batter on a food scale and divide by 10. That will give you the grams of batter per cup.

Crumble Topping

- Add walnuts, butter, and almond flour to food processor.

- Pulse a few times until nuts are chopped into small pieces. If mixture seems too dry (sometimes some walnuts are softer than others) feel free to add another tablespoon of butter.

- Sprinkle bits of the mixture evenly over batter and gently press down.

- Sprinkle erythritol on top of crumble mixture.

- Bake for 20 minutes or until golden and toothpick comes out clean. Let cool for at least 30 minutes, an hour or more if possible. This lets them firm up.

- *If they seem to be cooking faster, take them out sooner to avoid burning. Alternatively, if they are still wet looking, return them to the oven for a few minutes keeping a close eye on them.

Nutrition Info

Calories: 184

Total Carbs: 7g

Fiber: 3g

Net Carbs: 4g

Protein: 7g

Fat: 14g

Keto Fat Bombs

These fat bombs are your best friend. Don't let the name scare you—these little balls are the perfect way to curb your hunger.

Yields: 8
Prep Time: 0 hours 5 mins
Total Time: 0 hours 25 mins

Ingredients

- 8 oz. cream cheese, softened to room temperature
- 1/2 c. keto-friendly peanut butter
- 1/4 c. coconut oil, plus 2 tbsp.
- 1/2 tsp. kosher salt
- 1 c. keto-friendly dark chocolate chips (such as Lily's)

Instructions

- Line a small baking sheet with parchment paper. In a medium bowl, combine cream cheese, peanut butter, ¼ c coconut oil, and salt. Using a hand mixer, beat mixture until fully combined, about 2 minutes. Place bowl in freezer to firm up slightly, 10 to 15 minutes.

- When peanut butter mixture has hardened, use a small cookie scoop or spoon to create golf ball sized balls. Place in the refrigerator to harden, 5 minutes.
- Meanwhile, make chocolate drizzle: combine chocolate chips and remaining coconut oil in a microwave safe bowl and microwave in 30 second intervals until fully melted. Drizzle over peanut butter balls and place back in the refrigerator to harden, 5 minutes. Serve.
- To store, keep covered in refrigerator.

Nutrition Info

Per Serving: 84 calories; 8.4 g fat; 2.6 g carbohydrates; 2 g protein; 0 mg cholesterol; 0 mg sodium

Zucchini Egg Cups

Yields: 12
Prep Time: 0 hours 10 mins
Total Time: 0 hours 40 mins

Ingredients

- Cooking spray, for pan
- 2 zucchini, peeled into strips
- 1/4 lb. ham, chopped
- 1/2 c. cherry tomatoes, quartered
- 8 eggs
- 1/2 c. heavy cream
- Kosher salt
- Freshly ground black pepper
- 1/2 tsp. dried oregano
- 1 c. Pinch red pepper flakes
- 1 c. shredded cheddar

Instructions

- Preheat oven to 400° and grease a muffin tin with cooking spray. Line the inside and bottom of the muffin tin with zucchini strips, to form a crust. Sprinkle ham and cherry tomatoes inside each crust.

- In a medium bowl whisk together eggs, heavy, cream, oregano, and red pepper flakes then season with salt and pepper. Pour egg mixture over ham and tomatoes then top with cheese.
- Bake until eggs are set, 30 minutes.

Ham & Cheese Breakfast Roll-Ups

Yields: 2
Prep Time: 0 hours 20 mins
Total Time: 0 hours 20 mins

Ingredients

- 4 large eggs
- 1/4 c. milk
- 2 tbsp. Chopped chives
- kosher salt
- Freshly ground black pepper
- 1 tbsp. butter
- 1 c. shredded cheddar, divided
- 4 slices ham

Instructions

- In a medium bowl, whisk together eggs, milk, and chives. Season with salt and pepper.
- In a medium skillet over medium heat, melt butter. Pour half of the egg mixture into the skillet, moving to create a thin layer that covers the entire pan.
- Cook for 2 minutes. Add 1/2 cup cheddar and cover for 2 minutes more, until the

cheese is melty. Remove onto plate, place 2 slices of ham, and roll tightly. Repeat with remaining ingredients and serve.

Nutrition Info

Calories: 260
Fat: 21 g
Saturated Fat: 11 g
Trans Fat: 0.5 g
Sodium: 530 mg
Sugars: 1 g
Protein: 17 g
Fibre: 0 g
Carbohydrate: 0 g

Curry Tofu Scramble with Avocado

This tofu scramble is a fabulous low carb veggie lover approach to begin the morning, with a lot of supplements and sufficient calories togive you vitality for the day ahead.

Prep Time 5 minutes;
Cook Time 13 minutes;
Total Time 20 minutes,
Calories 380 kcal
Servings 3

Ingredients:

- 1 tbsp coconut oil
- 2 tbsp olive oil
- 300 g tofu (extra firm)
- 1 tsp turmeric
- 1 tbsp nutritional yeast
- 1 tbsp curry powder
- 1/2 cup zucchini (chopped)
- 1 cup mushrooms (chopped)
- 1 tomato (chopped)
- cilantro (optional)(to garnish)
- 300-gram avocado

Instructions

- The initial step is to dry the tofu so it ingests the flavor.
- Cut the tofu into 1 inch long strips, spread out the strips on a paper towel,
- put another paper towel to finish everything and after that a slashing board.
- Place something substantial over this, for example, a few books.
- Abandon it to sit for around 15 minutes.
- Add the coconut oil to the dish and disintegrate the tofu into the skillet with your hands.
- Cook for around 5 minutes, mixing every now and again.
- Include the turmeric, nourishing yeast and curry powder and 1 tbsp of the olive oil,
- blend and cook for a further 4 minutes.
- Add whatever remains of the olive oil, zucchini, mushroom and tomato and sear for a further 4 minutes blending much of the time.
- Serve with 1 little medium size avocado (roughly 100g) cut.

Recipe Notes:
This meal can be refrigerated for a few days.
Nutritional Information:
Calories: 381, Fats: 32g, Protein: 11g, Net Carbs: 8g

Avocado Egg Boats

Prep Time: 0 hours 10 mins
Total Time: 0 hours 30 mins

Ingredients

- 2 ripe avocados, pitted and halved
- 4 large eggs
- kosher salt
- Freshly ground black pepper
- 3 slices bacon
- Freshly chopped chives, for garnish

Instructions

- Preheat oven to 350°. Place avocados in a baking dish, then crack eggs into a bowl. Using a spoon, transfer yolks to each avocado half, then spoon in as much egg white as you can fit without spilling over.
- Season with salt and pepper and bake until whites are set and yolks are no longer runny, about 20 minutes. (Cover with foil if avocados are beginning to brown.)
- Meanwhile, in a large skillet over medium heat, cook bacon until crisp, 8 minutes, then

transfer to a paper towel-lined plate and chop.

- Top avocados with bacon and chives and serve with a spoon.

Nutrition Info

Calories 251

Keto Cannoli Stuffed Crepes

These Keto Cannoli Stuffed Crepes are perfect for any special occasion breakfast or brunch! Tastes like you're cheating, but they are low carb, gluten free, grain free, Atkins, and nut free too!

Prep Time: 15 minutes
Cook Time: 20 minutes
Total Time: 35 minutes
Yield: 4 servings

Ingredients

For the crepes:

- 8 ounces cream cheese, softened
- 8 eggs
- 1/2 teaspoon ground cinnamon
- 1 tablespoon granulated erythritol sweetener
- 2 tablespoons butter, for the pan

For the cannoli filling:

- 6 ounces mascarpone cheese, softened
- 1 cup whole milk ricotta cheese
- 1/2 teaspoon lemon zest

- 1/2 teaspoon ground cinnamon
- 1/4 teaspoon unsweetened vanilla extract
- 1/4 cup powdered erythritol sweetener

For the optional chocolate drizzle (not included in nutrition info:)

3 squares of a Lindt 90% chocolate bar

Instructions

For the crepes:

- Combine all of the crepes ingredients in a blender and blend until smooth.
- Let the batter rest for 5 minutes and then give it a stir to break up any additional air bubbles.
- Heat 1 teaspoon of butter in a 10 inch or larger nonstick saute pan over medium heat.
- When the butter is melted and bubbling, pour in about 1/4 cup of batter (you can eyeball it) and if necessary, gently tilt the pan in a circular motion to create a 6-inch (-ish) round crepe.
- Cook for two minutes, or until the top is no longer glossy and bubbles have formed almost to the middle of the crepe.
- Carefully flip and cook for another 30 seconds. Remove and place on a plate.
- Repeat until you have 8 usable crepes.

Nutrition Info

Serving Size: 2 stuffed crepes
Calories: 478
Fat: 42g
Carbohydrates: 4g
Fiber: 0g
Protein: 16g

Chocolate-Raspberry Chia Pudding Shots

Dessert and breakfast, together once more! These Chocolate-Raspberry Chia pudding shots are relatively similar to enchantment. They're solid and sweet - the ideal mix. Celebrated for being a low carb thickening agent, these natural chia seeds make a remarkable pudding!

Course: Breakfast, Dessert;
Prep Time 1 hour;
Servings 2; Calories 240 kcal

Ingredients:

- ¼ cup chia seeds
- 1/2 cup coconut milk
- 1/4 cup almond milk
- 1 tablespoon cacao powder
- 1 tablespoon Stevia
- 1/2 cup raspberries

Instructions:

- In a container, bring together all the ingredients (with the exception of the raspberries) and shake vivaciously. Let sit for 2 minutes and after that fill four shot glasses.

- Refrigerate for no less than 60 minutes (ideally across the night) until the point that blend thickens into pudding. Top with raspberries.

Recipe Notes:

This yield of this recipe is 4 shots. 1 serving is 2 shots.

Nutritional Information:
Calories: 241, Protein: 4g Fats: 20g, , Net Carbs: 4g

LUNCH

Keto Chicken Enchilada Bowl

This Keto Chicken Enchilada Bowl is a low carb twist on a Mexican favorite!

Prep Time: 20 minutes
Cook Time: 30 minutes
Total Time: 50 minutes
Yield: 4 servings

Ingredients

- 2 tablespoons coconut oil (for searing chicken)
- 1 pound of boneless, skinless chicken thighs
- 3/4 cup red enchilada sauce (recipe from Low Carb Maven)
- 1/4 cup water
- 1/4 cup chopped onion
- 4 oz can diced green chiles

Toppings (feel free to customize)

- 1 whole avocado, diced
- 1 cup shredded cheese (I used mild cheddar)

- 1/4 cup chopped pickled jalapenos
- 1/2 cup sour cream
- 1 roma tomato, chopped

Optional: serve over plain cauliflower rice (or Mexican cauliflower rice) for a more complete meal!

Instructions

- In a pot or dutch oven over medium heat melt the coconut oil. Once hot, sear chicken thighs until lightly brown.

- Pour in enchilada sauce and water then add onion and green chiles. Reduce heat to a simmer and cover. Cook chicken for 17-25 minutes or until chicken is tender and fully cooked through to at least 165 degrees internal temperature.

- Carefully remove the chicken and place onto a work surface. Chop or shred chicken (your preference) then add it back into the pot. Let the chicken simmer uncovered for an additional 10 minutes to absorb flavor and allow the sauce to reduce a little.

- To Serve, top with avocado, cheese, jalapeno, sour cream, tomato, and any other desired toppings. Feel free to customize these to your preference. Serve alone or over cauliflower rice if desired just be sure to update your personal nutrition info as needed.

Nutrition Info

Calories: 568 Calories

Total Carbs: 10.41g

Fiber: 4.27g

Net Carbs: 6.14g

Protein: 38.38g

Fat: 40.21g

Almond Coconut Curry on Veges

This almond coconut curry is super speedy and simple and tastes extraordinary as well! It flaunts nutritious vegetables alongside solid fats and a decent calorie tally.

Time 15 minutes; Total Time 15 minutes;
Servings 4; Calories 439 kcal

Ingredients:

For the veges
For the curry

- 1 tsp coconut oil
- 400 ml coconut milk
- 2 cups mushrooms
- 125 g almond butter (100% ground almonds)
- 4 cups spinach
- 1 tbsp tomato paste
- 2 cups brocolli (chopped into florets)
- 1 tbsp curry powder

Instructions:

For the curry mixture

- Put the coconut drain, almond spread, tomato glue and curry powder in a blender. Mix for around 20 seconds or until smooth.
- Add the curry blend to a pan on low-medium warmth and warmth for 10-15 minutes or until warmed through. Blend habitually to abstain from staying.

For the veges

- Heat the coconut oil in a container on medium-high warmth and include the broccoli and mushrooms. Sear for around 3 minutes. Include the spinach and warmth for one more moment.

- Serve the veges in a bowl with the curry blend poured over the best.

Recipe Notes:

You can make the almond margarine by granulating almonds in a sustenance processor.

The curry blend isolates whenever left to sit in the refrigerator for some time, so make certain to mix it completely before utilizing on the off chance that you have put away it in the ice chest.

Nutritional Information:
Calories: 438, Fats: 41g, Protein: 11g, Net Carbs: 9g

Sesame Salmon w. Baby Bok Choy & Mushrooms

Ingredients

Main Dish

- 4 each 4-6 oz. salmon fillet
- 2 each portobello mushroom caps (or 8 oz. baby bella mushrooms)
- 4 each baby bok choy
- 1 tbsp toasted sesame seeds
- 1 ea green onion

Marinade

- 1 tbsp olive oil
- 1 tsp sesame oil
- 1 tbsp Coconut Aminos
- 1/2 inch Ginger grated (approx. 1 tsp.)
- 1/2 lemon juice
- 1/2 tsp Salt
- 1/2 tsp black pepper

Instructions

- Whisk together all of your marinade ingredients
- Drizzle half of the marinade on the salmon and turn to coat. Cover and refrigerate the salmon while it marinates for one hour.
- Preheat oven to 400.
- Prepare vegetables: Trim the rough ends from the bok choy and cut into halves. Slice the mushrooms into ½ inch pieces.
- Drizzle the remaining marinade over the vegetables and lay on a lined baking sheet.
- Place salmon, skin side down, on a lined baking sheet as well. Bake until salmon is cooked through, about 20 minutes.
- Top with sliced green onions and sesame seeds.

Caprese Tuna Salad Stuffed Tomatoes

Prep Time: 10 minutes
Yield: Serves 1
Serving Size: entire recipe
Calories per serving: 196
Fat per serving: 4.9g

Ingredients

- 1 medium tomato
- 1 (5oz) can tuna, very well drained
- 2 tsp balsamic vinegar
- 1 TBSP chopped mozzarella {1/4 oz.}
- 1 TBSP chopped fresh basil
- 1 TBSP chopped green onion

Instructions

- Cut the top 1/4-inch off the tomato. Use a spoon to scoop out the insides of the tomato. Set aside while you make the tuna salad.
- Stir together the drained tuna, balsamic vinegar, mozzarella, basil, and green onion. Put the tuna salad in the hollowed out tomato, and enjoy!
- Note: I prefer using fresh mozzarella but any mozzarella is good in here.

Salmon & Avocado Nori Rolls (Paleo Sushi)

Prep time: 10 mins
Total time: 10 mins
Recipe type: Lunch
Serves: 1

Ingredients

- 3 square nori sheets (seaweed wrappers)
- 150-180 g / 5-6 oz cooked salmon or tinned salmon
- ⅓ red pepper, sliced into thin strips
- ½ avocado, sliced into strips
- ½ small cucumber, sliced into strips
- 1 spring onion/scallion, cut into 2-3" pieces
- 2 tablespoons mayonnaise
- 1 tablespoon hot sauce or Sriracha sauce
- 1 teaspoon black or white sesame seeds
- Coconut aminos for dipping, optional

Instructions

- Place the nori sheet on a flat surface, such as a cutting board, shiny side down. Look at the fibres of the wrapper to see which way it needs to be rolled.
- Add a third of the salmon to the right or left third of the nori sheet and top with two strips of pepper, cucumber and avocado. Add some green onion and a drizzle of mayonnaise and hot sauce. You can sprinkle with sesame seeds now or at a later stage, once the rolls are cut.
- Lightly wet the top part of the nori sheet (the side you are rolling towards), just 1-2 cm of the wrapper. Pick up the opposite outer edge of the roll and start wrapping it over the ingredients, using your fingers to keep it nice and tight. This can take a bit of practice, but don't worry if your roll doesn't look perfect. Roll it until the top edge of the wrapper overlaps the roll and press it tightly to stick. Place the roll on the cutting board with the seam facing down and then cut into bite-size pieces.
- Serve right away with some coconut aminos or extra mayo for dipping, or pack in a container to take for lunch or keep as a snack in the fridge.

Cinnamon Pork Chops & Mock Apples

Hearty, healthy, and delicious, cinnamon pork chops with chayote mock apples makes a fantastic family dinner or meal prep for the work week!

Prep Time 5 minutes
Cook Time 40 minutes
Total Time 45 minutes

Ingredients

- 2 tbsp ghee
- 1/2 tsp sea salt
- 4 pork chops boneless
- 2 chayote chopped to 1/2-inch chunks
- 2 tbsp monkfruit sweetener or low carb sweetener of choice
- 1 tsp cinnamon
- 1/8 tsp nutmeg
- 1 tbsp apple cider vinegar

Instructions

- Melt ghee in a large skillet over medium heat, add pork chops and cook for 5 minutes.

- Flip the pork chops and add chayote and sprinkle sweetener, cinnamon, nutmeg, and apple cider vinegar over the top. Cook for an additional 4-5 minutes, or until the pork chops reach the appropriate temperature (145 F for medium rare, 160 for medium).

- Remove the pork chops and place in a meal prep container if preparing meals for the week, otherwise keep pork chops warm until ready to serve.

- Bring the chayote mixture to a boil for several minutes. Reduce heat to low medium and simmer with cover, stirring occasionally, for 30 to 40 minutes. When done, the chayote will be fork tender and similar in texture to baked apple.

- Divide the chayote mock apples between four meal prep containers or serve immediately alongside the warm pork chops.

Recipe Notes

2g net carbohydrates per serving - which gives you room for a couple more things if you'd like to add that to your meal prep container or tailor things to your personal macros.

Nutritional Information:

Net Carbs: 4.85g
Protein: 35.43g
Fat: 30.22g
Calories: 455kcal

Loaded Chicken Salad

A delicious salad filled with plenty of vegetables and delicious grilled meat!

Prep Time 10 minutes
Cook Time 8 minutes
Total Time 18 minutes
Total Carbs 12.86g

Ingredients

- 1 boneless chicken breast (about 300g, with or without skin)
- 1 tbsp extra virgin olive oil
- 1/4 tsp Himalayan salt
- 1/4 tsp black pepper
- 1 avocado
- 100 g mozzarella balls
- 1 large tomato (any colour)
- 1 har artichoke hearts (my jar was 170g)
- 1/2 red onion
- 5 asparagus
- 20 leaves basil
- 4 cups baby spinach (200g used)

Dressing

- 2 tbsp extra virgin olive oil
- 1 1/2 tbsp balsamic vinegar
- 1 tsp dijon mustard
- 1 clove garlic
- pinch Himalayan salt
- pinch black pepper

Instructions

- Peel and dice the avocado. Slice the red onion. Dice the tomato. Pile the basil leaves together, roll them up and slice. Cut the stems off the asparagus and slice in half. Mince the garlic.
- Slice the chicken breast in half lengthwise. Sprinkle the 1/4 tsp of salt and pepper on each sides. Heat the 1 tbsp of olive oil in a cast iron skillet and place the chicken breasts in. Fry on each side, about 3 minutes each side, until they have a nice golden brown colour and cooked through. Add the asparagus beside the chicken breasts and cook a few minutes until soft and grilled. Take out the chicken and slice.

- In a small bowl, combine the minced garlic, olive oil, balsamic vinegar, dijon, and salt & pepper.
- Add the baby spinach to a large bowl or plate. Cover with the grilled chicken, avocado, mozzarella, tomatoes, artichoke, red onions, asparagus and basil leaves. Pour the dressing over and enjoy!

Notes

You can add 1 tbsp of honey to the salad dressing if you don't mind the extra carbs or want a sweeter dressing.

Nutrition Info

Calories 430 Calories from Fat 264

Saturated Fat 6.57g 33%

Total Carbohydrates 12.86g 4%

Dietary Fiber 6.12g 24%

Sugars 3.16g

Protein 31.73g 63%

Dinner and Desert

Keto Instant Pot Crack Chicken Recipe

Cuisine: American
Prep time: 5 mins
Cook time: 20 mins
Total time: 25 mins
Serves: 8 servings (yields about 7 cups total)

Rich, creamy, and full of flavor, this Keto Instant Pot Crack Chicken Recipe is sure to be a favorite family dinner.

Ingredients

- 2 slices bacon, chopped
- 2 lbs (910 g) boneless, skinless chicken breasts
- 2 (8 oz/227 g) blocks cream cheese
- ½ cup (120 ml) water
- 2 tablespoons apple cider vinegar
- 1 tablespoon dried chives
- 1½ teaspoons garlic powder
- 1½ teaspoons onion powder
- 1 teaspoon crushed red pepper flakes

- 1 teaspoon dried dill
- ¼ teaspoon salt
- ¼ teaspoon black pepper
- ½ cup (2 oz/57 g) shredded cheddar
- 1 scallion, green and white parts, thinly sliced

Instructions

- Turn pressure cooker on, press "Sauté", and wait 2 minutes for the pot to heat up. Add the chopped bacon and cook until crispy. Transfer to a plate and set aside. Press "Cancel" to stop sautéing.
- Add the chicken, cream cheese, water, vinegar, chives, garlic powder, onion powder, crushed red pepper flakes, dill, salt, and black pepper to the pot. Turn the pot on Manual, High Pressure for 15 minutes and then do a quick release.
- Use tongs to transfer the chicken to a large plate, shred it with 2 forks, and return it back to the pot.
- Stir in the cheddar cheese.
- Top with the crispy bacon and scallion, and serve.

Notes

We've tested this recipe upwards of 10 times and have never had the burn warning come on; however, several readers have had the warning come on, so we want to give a tip. In step 1 of the Instructions above, after removing the bacon from the pot, we recommend adding a splash of water, and use a wooden spoon to scrape up any brown bits that have formed on the bottom to deglaze the pan. After that, continue on with step 1 and press "Cancel" to stop sauteing.

Nutrition Facts

Calories: 437 Fat: 27.6 Potassium: 390 Net Carbs: 4.3 Carbohydrates: 4.5 Sodium: 420 Fiber: .2 Protein: 41.2

Keto Chicken Enchilada Bowl

This Keto Chicken Enchilada Bowl is a low carb twist on a Mexican favorite! It's So easy to make, totally filling and ridiculously yummy!

Prep Time: 20 minutes
Cook Time: 30 minutes
Total Time: 50 minutes
Yield: 4 servings

Ingredients

- 2 tablespoons coconut oil (for searing chicken)
- 1 pound of boneless, skinless chicken thighs
- 3/4 cup red enchilada sauce (recipe from Low Carb Maven)
- 1/4 cup water
- 1/4 cup chopped onion
- 4 oz can diced green chiles

Toppings (feel free to customize)

- 1 whole avocado, diced
- 1 cup shredded cheese (I used mild cheddar)
- 1/4 cup chopped pickled jalapenos

- 1/2 cup sour cream
- 1 roma tomato, chopped

Optional: serve over plain cauliflower rice (or mexican cauliflower rice) for a more complete meal!

Instructions

- In a pot or dutch oven over medium heat melt the coconut oil. Once hot, sear chicken thighs until lightly brown.

- Pour in enchilada sauce and water then add onion and green chiles. Reduce heat to a simmer and cover. Cook chicken for 17-25 minutes or until chicken is tender and fully cooked through to at least 165 degrees internal temperature.

- Careully remove the chicken and place onto a work surface. Chop or shred chicken (your preference) then add it back into the pot. Let the chicken simmer uncovered for an additional 10 minutes to absorb flavor and allow the sauce to reduce a little.

- To Serve, top with avocado, cheese, jalapeno, sour cream, tomato, and any other desired toppings. Feel free to customize these to your preference. Serve alone or over cauliflower rice if desired just be sure to update your personal nutrition info as needed.

Nutrition Info

Calories: 568 Calories
Total Carbs: 10.41g
Fiber: 4.27g
Net Carbs: 6.14g
Protein: 38.38g
Fat: 40.21g

Crab Stuffed Mushrooms With Cream Cheese

An easy recipe for crab stuffed mushrooms with cream cheese. Low carb, keto, and gluten free.

Prep Time 15 minutes
Cook Time 30 minutes
Servings 4 servings
Calories 160 kcal

Ingredients

- 20 ounces cremini (baby bella) mushrooms (20-25 individual mushrooms)
- 2 tablespoons finely grated parmesan cheese
- 1 tablespoon chopped fresh parsley
- salt

Filling:

- 4 ounces cream cheese softened to room temperature
- 4 ounces crab meat finely chopped
- 5 cloves garlic minced
- 1 teaspoon dried oregano
- 1/2 teaspoon paprika

- 1/2 teaspoon black pepper
- 1/4 teaspoon salt

Instructions

- Preheat the oven to 400 F. Prepare a baking sheet lined with parchment paper.
- Snap stems from mushrooms, discarding the stems and placing the mushroom caps on the baking sheet 1 inch apart from each other. Season the mushroom caps with salt.
- In a large mixing bowl, combine all filling ingredients and stir until well-mixed without any lumps of cream cheese. Stuff the mushroom caps with the mixture. Evenly sprinkle parmesan cheese on top of the stuffed mushrooms.
- Bake at 400 F until the mushrooms are very tender and the stuffing is nicely browned on top, about 30 minutes. Top with parsley and serve while hot.

Nutrition Notes

This recipe yields 5 g net carbs per serving (5-6 stuffed mushrooms).

Nutrition Info

Calories 160
Total Carb 5.5g 2%
Dietary Fiber 0.5g 1%
Sugars 0g
Protein 9g

Lemon Butter Sauce for Fish

Prep: 5 mins
Cook: 10 mins
Total: 15 mins

A Lemon Butter Sauce with Crispy Pan Fried Fish that would be perfectly at home in a posh restaurant, yet is so ⬚uick to make at home! Browning the butter gives the sauce a rich, nutty aroma which pairs beautifully with fresh lemon, as well as thickening the sauce and giving it a gorgeous golden colour. Recipe VIDEO below (helpful for pre-post browned butter).

Servings: 2
Calories: 393 kcal

Ingredients

Lemon Butter Sauce:

- 60 g / 4 tbsp unsalted butter, cut into pieces
- 1 tbsp fresh lemon juice
- Salt and finely ground pepper

Crispy Pan Fried Fish:

- 2 x thin white fish fillets (120-150g / 4-5oz each), skinless boneless (I used Bream, Note 1)
- Salt and pepper
- 2 tbsp white flour
- 2 tbsp oil (I use canola)

Serving:

- Lemon wedges
- Finely chopped parsley, optional

Instructions

- Lemon Butter Sauce (see video):

- Place the butter in a light coloured saucepan or small skillet over medium heat.

- Melt butter then leave on the stove, whisking / stirring very now and then. When the butter turns golden brown and it smells nutty - about 3 minutes, remove from stove immediately and pour into small bowl. (Note 2)

- Add lemon juice and a pinch of salt and pepper. Stir then taste when it has cooled slightly. Adjust lemon/salt to taste.

- Set aside - it will stay pourable for 20 - 30 minutes. See Note 3 for storing.

Crispy Pan Fried Fish:

- Pat fish dry using paper towels. Sprinkle with salt & pepper, then flour. Use fingers to spread flour. Turn and repeat. Shake excess flour off well, slapping between hands if necessary.

- Heat oil in a nonstick skillet over high heat. When the oil is shimmering and there are faint wisps of smoke, add fish. Cook for 1 1/2 minutes until golden and crispy on the edges, then turn and cook the other side for 1 1/2 minutes (cook longer if you have thicker fillets).

- Remove immediately onto serving plates. Drizzle each with about 1 tbsp of Sauce (avoid dark specks settled at the bottom of the bowl), garnish with parsley and serve with lemon on the side. Pictured in post with Kale and Quinoa Salad.

Recipe Notes

If you're an experienced cook, you can try your hand at making the sauce in the pan after cooking the fish. First wipe it clean (yes you lose pan flavour, but it's nice to have a "clean" looking sauce), lower heat then make the sauce once the pan has cooled. I personally find it easier to make the Sauce first in a smaller pan - easier to control colour change. Also I like using my black non stick pan for the fish and you can't see the colour of the butter in dark coloured pans.

Easy Tomato Feta Soup Recipe

Prep Time:5 mins
Cook Time:25 mins
Total Time:30 mins
Servings: 6

Easy Tomato Feta Soup Recipe - Low Calorie, Low Carb, Keto - simple to make with just a few simple basic ingredients. Creamy tomato soup with basil and rich, savory feta cheese. Ready on 30 minutes on the stove top.

Ingredients

- 2 tbsp olive oil or butter
- 1/4 cup chopped onion
- 2 cloves garlic
- 1/2 tsp salt
- 1/8 tsp black pepper
- 1 tsp pesto sauce — optional
- 1/2 tsp dried oregano
- 1 tsp dried basil
- 1 tbsp tomato paste — optional
- 10 tomatoes, skinned, seeded and chopped — or two 14.5 oz cans of peeled tomatoes
- 1 tsp honey, sugar or erythritol — optional
- 3 cups water
- 1/3 cup heavy cream
- 2/3 cup feta cheese — crumbled

Instructions

- Heat olive oil (butter) over medium heat in a large pot (Dutch Oven). Add the onion and cook for 2 minutes, stirring frequently. Add the garlic and cook for 1 minute. Add tomatoes, salt, pepper, pesto (optional), oregano, basil, tomato paste and water. Bring to a boil, then reduce to a simmer. Add sweetener.

- Cook on medium heat for 20 minutes, until the tomatoes are tender and cooker. Using an immersion blender, blend until smooth. Add the cream and feta cheese. Cook for 1 more minute.

- Add more salt if needed. Serve warm.

Recipe Notes

For people who are against using heavy cream in keto diet, you can use almond milk.

Nutrition Information

Calories: 170, Fat: 13g, Saturated Fat: 8g, Cholesterol: 43mg, Sodium: 464mg, Potassium: 542mg, Carbohydrates: 10g, Fiber: 2g, Sugar: 6g, Protein: 4g, Vitamin A: 43%, Vitamin C: 35.7%, Calcium: 11.9%, Iron: 4.9%

Instant Pot Beef Bourguignon

Instant Pot Beef Bourguignon is a pressure cooker recipe with beef, mushrooms, onions, and carrots cooked in red wine. Low carb, keto, and gluten free.

Prep Time 30 minutes
Cook Time 50 minutes
Servings 6 servings
Calories 220 kcal

Ingredients

- 1.5 - 2 pounds beef chuck roast cut into 3/4-inch cubes
- 5 strips bacon diced
- 1 small onion chopped
- 10 ounces cremini mushrooms quartered
- 2 carrots chopped
- 5 cloves garlic minced
- 3 bay leaves
- 3/4 cup dry red wine
- 3/4 teaspoon xanthan gum (or corn starch, read post for instructions)
- 1 tablespoon tomato paste
- 1 teaspoon dried thyme
- salt & pepper

Instructions

- Generously season beef chunks with salt and pepper, and set aside. Select the saute mode on the pressure cooker for medium heat. When the display reads HOT, add diced bacon and cook for about 5 minutes until crispy, stirring fre uently. Transfer the bacon to a paper towel lined plate.

- Add the beef to the pot in a single layer and cook for a few minutes to brown, then flip and repeat for the other side. Transfer to a plate when done.

- Add onions and garlic. Cook for a few minutes to soften, stirring frequently. Add red wine and tomato paste, using a wooden spoon to briefly scrape up flavorful brown bits stuck to the bottom of the pot. Stir to check that the tomato paste is dissolved. Turn off the saute mode.

- Transfer the beef back to the pot. Add mushrooms, carrots, and thyme, stirring together. Top with bay leaves. Secure and seal the lid. Cook at high pressure for 40 minutes, followed by a manual pressure release.

- Uncover and select the saute mode. Remove bay leaves. Evenly sprinkle xanthan gum over the pot and stir together. Let the stew boil for a minute to thicken while stirring. Turn off the saute mode. Serve into bowls and top with crispy bacon.

Nutrition Notes

This recipe yields 5.5 g net carbs per serving (1-1.5 cups).

Nutrition Info

Calories 220
Total Fat 5g 8%
Sodium 310mg 13%
Potassium 130mg 4%
Total Carb 6.5g 2%
Dietary Fiber 1g 3%
Sugars 2g
Protein 27g

Keto Chicken Pot Pie

Cook Time22 mins
Course: Main Course
Servings: 8 servings
Calories: 297kcal

Ingredients

For the Chicken Pot Pie Filling:

- 2 tablespoons of butter
- 1/2 cup mixed veggies could also substitute green beans or broccoli
- 1/4 small onion diced
- 1/4 tsp pink salt
- 1/4 tsp pepper
- 2 garlic cloves minced
- 3/4 cup heavy whipping cream
- 1 cup chicken broth
- 1 tsp poultry seasoning
- 1/4 tsp rosemary
- pinch thyme
- 2 1/2 cups cooked chicken diced
- 1/4 tsp Xanthan Gum

For the crust:

- 4 1/2 tablespoons of butter melted and cooled
- 1/3 cup coconut flour
- 2 tablespoons full fat sour cream
- 4 eggs
- 1/4 teaspoon salt
- 1/4 teaspoon baking powder
- 1 1/3 cup sharp shredded cheddar cheese or mozzarella shredded

Instructions

- Cook 1 to 1 1/2 lbs chicken in the slow cooker for 3 hours on high or 6 hours on low.
- Preheat oven to 400 degrees.
- Sautee onion, mixed veggies, garlic cloves, salt, and pepper in 2 tablespoons butter in an oven safe skillet for approx 5 min or until onions are translucent.
- Add heavy whipping cream, chicken broth, poultry seasoning, thyme, and rosemary.
- Sprinkle Xanthan Gum on top and simmer for 5 minutes so that the sauce thickens. Make sure to simmer covered as the liquid will evaporate otherwise. You need a lot of

liquid for this recipe, otherwise, it will be dry.

- Add diced chicken.
- Make the breading by combining melted butter (I cool mine by popping the bowl in the fridge for 5 min), eggs, salt, and sour cream in a bowl then whisk together.
- Add coconut flour and baking powder to the mixture and stir until combined.
- Stir in cheese.
- Drop batter by dollops on top of the chicken pot pie. Do not spread it out, as the coconut flour will absorb too much of the liquid.
- Bake in a 400-degree oven for 15-20 min.
- Set oven to broil and move chicken pot pie to top shelf. Broil for 1-2 minutes until bread topping is nicely browned.

Nutrition

Calories: 297kcal | Carbohydrates: 5.3g | Protein: 11.6g | Fat: 17g | Fiber: 2g

Easy Stir Fry Kimchi & Pork Belly

Stir-fry kimchi and bork belly is so simple to make yet out of this world satisfying! Dinner under 30 minutes, and Keto friendly.

Prep Time5 mins
Cook Time: 15 mins
Marinating: Time10 mins
Total Time: 20 mins
Servings: 3 people
Calories: 804 kcal

Ingredients

- 300 g naturally-raised pork belly
- 1 tbsp naturally-brewed tamari or soy sauce (gluten-free option: use tamari or gluten-free soy sauce)
- 1 tbsp naturally-brewed rice wine
- 1 lb kimchi (see notes below)
- 1 stalk green onion
- 1 tbsp sesame seeds (optional)

Instructions

- Slice the pork belly as thin as possible. Marinate in tamari/soy sauce and rice wine for about 10 minutes. If your kimchi isn't pre-cut, then cut into 1 inch size.

- Heat a heavy bottom pan (I use cast iron). While the pan is very hot, add the marinated pork belly, stir fry until nicely browned, for approximately 5 to 10 minutes. You should see some fat being cooked out of the pork belly at this point.

- Add the kimchi into the pan, stir-fry for another 2 minutes, for the flavour of kimchi and pork to completely mix.

- Turn off the heat. Thinly slice the green onion, and add to the stir fry.

- If available, sprinkle sesame seeds on top as garnish.

Recipe Notes

If you use a store-bought kimchi, make sure to check the ingredients. I use a home-made fermented kimchi that's free of MSG and added sugar (recipe coming soon.)

Spinach Artichoke Stuffed Chicken Breast Recipe

Spinach Artichoke Stuffed Chicken Breast is the perfect combination of your favorite dip and favorite bird, all rolled into one quick and easy Ketogenic stuffed chicken breast recipe! These spinach and mozzarella stuffed chicken breasts are gluten-free, low-carb, and Keto diet-approved!

Prep Time 15 minutes
Cook Time 15 minutes
Total Time 30 minutes
Servings 6 servings
Calories 288 kcal

Ingredients

- 1 ½ lbs. chicken breasts 6 4-oz. portions
- 2 tablespoons olive oil
- 4 ounces cream cheese softened
- ¼ cup Greek yogurt
- ½ cup Mozzarella cheese shredded
- ½ cup artichoke hearts thinly sliced
- ¼ cup frozen spinach drained, and tightly packed
- ½ tsp. salt divided
- ¼ tsp. pepper divided

Instructions

- Pound chicken breast to 1-inch thick. Using a sharp knife cut each chicken breast down the middle, being careful not to cut all of the way through, to make a pocket for the spinach artichoke filling. Sprinkle chicken breasts with ¼ teaspoon salt and 1/8 teaspoon pepper.
- In a medium-sized bowl combine the cream cheese, Greek yogurt, Mozzarella cheese, artichoke hearts, drained spinach, ¼ teaspoon salt and 1/8 teaspoon pepper. Mix until thoroughly combined.
- Carefully fill each chicken breast with equal amounts of the spinach artichoke filling. If you have extra filling, set it aside until the chicken is almost done cooking.
- In a large skillet over medium heat add olive oil and stuffed chicken breasts. Cover skillet and cook for 7-8 minutes on each side, or until chicken reaches 165 degrees with a meat thermometer.
- During the last few minutes of cooking, add additional filling to the skillet to heat it up. Serve chicken with cauliflower rice, regular rice, mashed cauliflower, or mashed potatoes and enjoy!

Nutrition Facts

Calories 288 Calories from Fat 153
Total Fat 17g 26%
Total Carbohydrates 2g 1%
Sugars 1g

CONCLUSION

The keto plan is a versatile and interesting way to lose weight, with lots of delicious food choices. Keep these 10 items stocked in your fridge, freezer, and larder, and you'll be ready to throw together some delicious keto meals and snacks at a moment's notice.